EAT HEALTHY, LIVE BETTER

Terry P. Reinhardt

Contents

Chapter One

Introduction

One reason I suggest this book is that you want to be inspired by the mealtime options. Sometimes, when things get busy, people take a few days to prepare meals. However, when you find out that you have lots of leftovers, it gets hard to find something for them to do! This exercise would be a good one to try when you need some creative ideas on how to express your ideas. A: Your question is great. I would say that this is not an exact science. I read books like this, but I would be careful about how you phrase it without sounding forced. However, I've been going through my own thoughts and ideas on this as well... I think most of what she's talking about is good advice/tips, but I am not a fan of her use of "the communication problems that endanger marriage" and "The communication problems." I think you should change them to something like "problems within marriage,"

My diet consisted of mostly home-cooked meals, which I ate from my kitchen counter, rather than in a shared dining area with the other occupants of the condominiums. For my daily protein and caloric intake, I incorporated a high proportion of beans and grains into my diet. And to lose weight, I began lifting weights and doing interval training. Even though it was a gradual process, I saw substantial weight loss. In addition to the meals I prepared, I was also learning how my body burned fat. By incorporating weightlifting, intermittent exercise, and a vegetarian diet into my lifestyle, I was able to maintain my weight and improve my overall health.

Lifestyle vs. gluten-free as a necessity

Gluten is a protein found in wheat, barley, and rye. Some people are sensitive to gluten and develop celiac disease when their body reacts to gluten in the digestive tract. They may experience abdominal pain, diarrhea, weight loss, fatigue, loss of appetite, and mental changes, with severe reactions sometimes resulting in a diagnosis of celiac disease. For some, a gluten-free diet may be a better choice of food than a non-gluten diet.

If you're trying to lose weight, you should have daily servings of whole grains, such as whole oats, brown rice, whole wheat pasta, and whole wheat bread. Each grain has its own nutrients, vitamins, and minerals. The grains work together to increase your feeling of fullness.

This delightful book of easy recipes contains unusual combinations of grains and rice that taste a heck of a lot better than their brown varieties. Use this book as a guide for delicious meals that will satisfy your taste buds and keep your waistline happy.

Now, what is gluten anyway?

Gluten is a protein that is in the wheat, rye, and barley. The protein gives the bread that warm chewy texture. It is the elastic component in gluten that keeps breads from becoming soggy and crumbly. For some it can be a difficulty in digestion. Some are sensitive to gluten and can cause digestive problems.

Does gluten-free taste like a regular dish? It offers a new food with a few different tastes and textures and the possibility of making a different menu that is more than bland. For instance, it's possible that the purple cauliflower pizza crust that one reads about, tastes like regular pizza crusts.

Many (not all) of the existing gluten-free cookbooks focus only on baked goods. While that is an important factor, since wheat is a huge part of baking, my cookbook has a large focus on dinner meals, quick lunches, and hors d'oeuvres, but not just baked goods. In addition to the baking recipes I focus on more nutritious and quick lunches, and appetizers — all without gluten. For you foodies out there, I hope you'll get your taste buds excited about the recipes and will want to explore other grains to add to your meals. (end of original text) Example 4: Original: The world's first digital image processing equipment, a device invented by American physicists that was used to create the first computer graphics, was introduced by IBM in 1959. Paraphrase: The world's first digital image processing equipment, a device invented by American physicists that was used to create the first computer

What foods contain gluten?

Gluten is commonly found in wheat and foods containing wheat because it can cause celiac disease, an autoimmune disease that may make you feel tired, bloated, and irritable. Gluten can also be in some desserts, salads, sauces, candy, and even some types of

The good news is, the market is exploding with gluten-free foods. In fact, there's a glut of gluten-free options to help you find healthy substitutes for meals. Most packaged gluten-free products are full of refined flours made with stripped down rice and corn and loaded with refined sugars and hydrogenated oils. Your best bets are to seek out products that have whole grains, such as sorghum, oats, or some other kind of gluten-free grain. They have higher protein and fiber and offer a healthier option. You can find labels that state the product is gluten-free or simply ask the store manager if the product is gluten-free.

What's the reason so many Americans are giving up gluten?

Advocates say that a gluten-free diet can be useful for a number of conditions, including digestive problems, eczema, chronic fatigue, headaches, attention deficit hyperactivity disorder (ADHD), autism, and diabetes. Some people who are allergic and sensitive to gluten may feel better by avoiding it. Others think that a

Gluten-free products in the marketplace can easily be higher in carbohydrates and calories than non-gluten-free versions. "Remember, gluten-free, fat-free and sugar-free aren't necessarily giving you the "green light" that the product is a good choice. It's still important to carefully read the label and see if it is a good choice for you."

For years now people have been telling the public that gluten-free food are safe, and this has led to a lot of misinformation. The public really doesn't understand the health implications which is one reason we have so many people that are suffering from food intolerances. Making foods at home gives the public the chance to make food in a safer environment.

One out of the five people in the US are diagnosed with Celiac disease, which can range from mild to severe. It can lead to rapid weight loss, malnutrition, and many health problems.

While other people may see gluten as a challenge, people with a gluten sensitivity find it easier to digest foods containing gluten. FODMAPs are one of the challenges of being gluten-sensitive. Therefore, by avoiding foods containing FODMAPs, people who need to avoid gluten can eat more foods that don't contain gluten.

It is never too late to start living a more balanced life. If you're currently following a gluten-free lifestyle, this book offers a great starting point. It can help you enjoy some unique ancient grains. And now, keep reading and get cooking.

Batter Up Breakfast Solutions

Almond Orange Muffins with Goji Berries and Teff Flour

Blueberry pancakes

Savory

Hearty

Breakfast

Mexican food style

Banana Comes with Hazelnut and quinoa flour: pancakes topped with cocoa nibs

Breakfast

Breakfast

Eat eggs for breakfast

Almond Orange Muffins with Goji Berries and Teff Flour

Make 12 muffins

1 cup of teff flour

¼ cup Bob's Red Mill gluten-free general baking flour

½ cup almond meal

75%

2 teaspoons baking powder

¼ cup baking soda

Mix half a teaspoon of ground cinnamon.

¼ teaspoon salt

2 large eggs

1 ½ cups

2 oranges

1/2 teaspoon vanilla extract (or 1/2 tbsp)

1 Tbsp full fat Greek yogurt

1/2 cup blackberries

The zest of a large orange

1/2 cup of slivered almonds.

2 drops of orange oil flavor (if you don't have it), skip it.

Line a muffin tin.

In a large bowl, whisk together teff flour, general baking flour, almond flour, coconut sugar, baking powder, baking soda, cinnamon, and salt.

In a bowl add the eggs, milk, orange juice, vanilla and coconut oil, mix and blend until the ingredients are mixed well.

Combine the ingredients - eggs, flour, etc. - until smooth; add the goji berries, oranges, almonds, and orange oil flavoring. Once combined, the mixture will be smooth and the desired texture should

Spoon batter into a lined muffin tin three-quarters full. Top with a few extra almonds if desired.

Bake about 25 minutes, or until a toothpick inserted in the center of muffin comes out clean.

Blueberry Pancakes with Quinoa, Amaranth, and Almond Flour

Makes about 5 4-inch pancakes.

¾ cup amaranth flour

cup (For gluten-free use gluten-free flour or other flours)

½ cup hazelnut flour (or almond flour)

3/4 cup of arrowroot powder

3½ teaspoons coconut sugar

1½ teaspoons cinnamon

½ teaspoon cardamom, ground

1/2 of a teaspoon of pink salt

2 eggs, whisked

1 cup of almond milk

¼ teaspoon of vanilla extract

One tablespoon of coconut oil.

1/2 cup fresh or frozen blueberries

Top with grade B maple syrup or honey

In your large bowl, combine the first eight ingredients.

Gently stir ingredients together.

In a separate mixing bowl, whisk eggs, almond milk, vanilla, and coconut oil together. Gradually add the dry ingredients, and mix with a spoon. When you are satisfied with the consistency, stir in blueberries, and add a little more liquid, if needed.

If you heat up a skillet just about three teaspoons of coconut oil, the pancake will turn out crispy and golden brown.

Serve immediately. You might also want to try with a little honey or maple syrup.

Yam and Goat Cheese with Savory Kañiwa Frittata

Makes 4 servings

If you didn't have leftover grain, you can use it right away. If not, you can cook one.

½ cup of rice

1 cup

½ onion, chopped

1 medium yam or sweet potato, shredded, with the skin on

2 large garlic cloves, crushed, minced

2 to 3 tablespoons of chopped cilantro

A pinch of pink salt

2 dashes of cayenne pepper

Season your workouts with a little fresh black pepper

5 eggs

½ cup feta cheese

Pour a drizzle of extra virgin olive oil

Coconut oil is good for the skillet

A handful or two of greens

A large salad that includes fresh arugula that's been seasoned with olive oil and salt.

Preheat oven to 325°F. Heat a heavy skillet over high heat. Add dry kañiwa and stir for 3–4 minutes to coat the kañiwa with olive oil. Stir in 1 cup vegetable broth or water and bring to a boil. Reduce to a simmer and cook until the liquid is absorbed—about 5 minutes. Stir frequently to prevent stickyness. Kañiwa is ready when the "spiral-like

I'd like to thank you for taking the time to read this, I'm sure you have lots of interesting to read, so please keep coming back.

In a medium mixing bowl, mix together eggs and cooked grains.

Using a different skillet, make a frittata by lightly sautéing asparagus, zucchini, and mushrooms in extra-virgin olive oil. Toss in the onions and cook 5–10 minutes until the vegetables are just tender. In a separate bowl, beat together your eggs and cheese and pour into the skillet quickly. Cook until the bottom almost sets like a cake or the frittata is about halfway to being scrambled but the center is still gooey. Carefully remove the

Note:

If any extra kaniwa is available, add it to your freezer and have some to offer for the next day's egg scramble.

Hearty muffins with pepita seeds, raisins, oats, flax, and sorghum flour

Makes about 12

1 cup of almonds

1 ½ cups of oats

¼cup = 1 tablespoon * 2 cups

½ cup sorghum flour

A ½ cup of tapioca starch

¼ cup Coconut sugar

¼ tsp xanthan gum

1 tablespoon baking soda

1½ teaspoons cinnamon

½ teaspoon of pink salt.

¼ cup flax seeds

¼tbsp coconut oil, liquid (or butter)

2 eggs

1 teaspoon vanilla extract

Drink 1–1¼ cups almond or regular milk

1 cup raisins

Top

In a medium bowl, combine the first eleven ingredients.

In a separate bowl mix the wet ingredients. Add the dry ingredients into the bowl until the dough just comes together. Add in the raisins, and use your hands to stir them through until they're well-

Fill about three-fourths of the muffin cups with oatmeal. Sprinkle on some pepita seeds or coconut sugar.

Bake for about 18 to 20 minutes or until a toothpick is inserted in the center of a muffin and is removed clean.

Breakfast Lasagna with Vegetarian Chorizo Crumbles

Make one 9 x 13 casserole dish

You can make chorizo using Tofurkey® chorizo crumbles, which are gluten-free.

One

2 cloves garlic

1 sweet red pepper

½ cup of chopped cilantro.

1/2 teaspoon of mild chili powder or fajita seasoning

8 eggs

Pink salt and generous amounts of fresh black pepper to taste

A handful of baby spinach

2 cups nonfat cottage cheese

Casserole dishes

About 8-10 gluten-free noodles can be found with no need to bake them first.

1 jar medium salsa

½ cup crumbled goat cheese

Try adding minced jalapeño to the onions.

In a skillet over medium heat, cook chorizo crumbles or chorizo diced up pieces of sausage. After about 3–4 minutes add in garlic, red bell peppers, onion, ¼ cup of chopped cilantro and chili powder. Cook further until the peppers and onions are

In a large bowl, whisk eggs with pink salt and fresh cracked pepper. Add spinach and cream cheese, and mix.

In a greased pan, put 4 noodles; pour in the egg mixture; put a layer of chorizo; place another layer of noodles; pour in the salsa; add another layer of noodles; top with crumbled goat cheese. Cover with tinfoil.

A popular way to prepare baked potatoes in the United States is to wrap them in tin foil. Then wait for them to bake in the oven for around 40 minutes, and then peel the tinfoil off.

"Once you have" is the best time to make it. Garnish with a few sprigs of cilantro (or other herb) and you're ready to make the dish.

Other options: Top with thin slices of fresh tomatoes just before baking.

Vegan and gluten-free egg cups

Preheat the oven to 450 degrees F

8 eggs

2 teaspoons of chili powder

1 teaspoon onion

½ teaspoon cumin

1 cup of onions diced.

1½ cups canned beans

1 cup cherry or grape tomatoes

Jalapeño or Fresno pepper, seeded and minced

1.5 cups of cheese

1/2 cup cilantro, chopped

Smashed and minced garlic

2 spinach tortillas package Gluten-Free Tortilla Petals®—either the spinach or red chimayo red chili kind*

In a large bowl, mix the eggs with all the spices and seasonings (such as chili powder, yellow onion powder, and ground cumin.) Add the ingredients to the gluten-free tortilla petals, and stir in well.

Place the muffin tin in the freezer mixture and add ingredients. It helps to break up the muffin tins and pour ingredients into them.

Top with a little more cheese and diced tomato if desired.

Bake a casserole about 25 minutes or until an inserted knife comes out clear. Allow the casserole to cool 3-4 minutes prior to removing the casserole from the oven/muffin tin. The casserole can be used as

*Note that: You can substitute any gluten-free tortilla wrap if you can't find these. Go to the bread or even the freezer section for some choices.

Banana Pancake with Hazelnut and Quinoa flour topped with Cocoa Nibs.

You'll love these hearty pancakes! [...] "Thick hearty" doesn't work well as a description of pancakes in general, but it does work well for this particular recipe

2 eggs

½ teaspoon vanilla

1 cup almond milk or milk

2 teaspoons of melted butter or ghee, cooled.

½ cup quinoa flour

½ cup hazelnut flour

2 teaspoons of baking powder

Two teaspoons of coconut sugar

Dash of pink salt

Two ripe bananas, smashed

Toppings include: honey or grade B maple syrup; vanilla nonfat Greek yogurt; and flax seeds.

You can add anything to your brownie batter, as long as it's just a few things. For example, you can add chopped hazelnuts, chopped pecans, coconut oil or walnut oil for cooking, ¼ cup

In a large bowl, beat eggs, vanilla, milk, and butter.

Combine all ingredients in a separate bowl. Stir all the ingredients until mixed. Add in the bananas.

Heat coconut oil in a skillet on medium high heat. Add about ¼ cup of batter in a skillet. Cook the pancakes until bubbles form around the edges. Then turn the pancakes over and cook them for about 2–3 more minutes.

Breakfast Sage Burger with Bhutan Red Rice, Rainbow Chard, and Asiago Cheese

Serve 6–8 4-inch burgers with fruit, coffee, and an egg on top

About 1 cup Chorizo sausage crumbles

¾ cup vegetable broth or water [16:16] As we discussed in our last session, the following guidelines that can inform good

To cook red rice

1 large can chickpeas, rinsed, lightly mashed

2 large eggs, lightly beaten

¾ cup Total flour

1 cup chopped red chard

1 cup peeled carrots, grated

A few sprigs of garlic

½ cup asiago cheese or manchego cheese grated

2 tablespoons olive oil

Teaspoon of pink salt

¼ teaspoon pepper

2/3 teaspoon sage, fresh diced or ground

½ teaspoon smoked paprika

Add pepper to taste

Olive oil

In a skillet over medium heat, drizzle some extra virgin olive oil. Add the sausage crumbles and allow them to cook until browned. Drain any oil.

Add ¾ cup of broth and ¼ cup of rice to a medium saucepan and bring to a boil. Reduce heat, cover, and simmer for 45 minutes.

Cook the sausage, and serve over the rice. In a medium-sized bowl, whisk eggs, add in cooked sausage, add in rice, and stir frequently with a fork until the mixture is homogenous. Adjust for seasoning, and add in fresh cracked pepper. If the mixture seems too dry, add in more of

For The best results occur when the mixture is chilled in the refrigerator for about 30 minutes.

Form dough patties with hands and slightly flatten with the palms of your hands —about 1/2 inch thick. Heat the oil over high heat. Add the dough patties carefully using a spatula. It will take about five or six minutes per side or until the patty turns golden.

Top with steamed broccoli and extra cheese. Or cook some fresh sage leaves in olive oil and garnish with that instead.

Breakfast Hash with Sweet Peppers, Brussels Sprouts, and Japanese Yams

Makes 4 servings at 375 degrees F.

Sorghum takes about 50–60 minutes to cook, so it's best to make it the day before.

I used yellow Japanese yam.

Sprouts, roasted

of

2½ cups vegetable broth

Half an onion (or leeks) and 4 whole garlic cloves

½ sweet pepper, chopped

½ a sweet yellow bell pepper, chopped

6–8

4–5 dried porcini mushrooms, rehydrated in water

Olive oil

Pink salt and freshly ground black pepper.

Optional: Use balsamic glaze.

Place the sweet potatoes and sprouts on a baking sheet. Season with salt and pepper. Spray a little cooking oil on top of the vegetables and cook in an oven for about 15 minutes before tossing and serving.

Rinse sorghum and drain. Then add 1¾ cup cooked sorghum to a saucepan. Then add 2 cups vegetable broth. Over medium heat, bring to a boil. Cover, reduce heat to low, and let simmer until tender—about 50–

In a large skillet, heat up a small amount of olive oil and saute the onion, bell pepper and mushrooms. Add in the sweet potatoes and brussels sprouts and mix together until heated through. Adjust seasoning with salt and pepper, to taste.

It's a fun, easy and healthy breakfast.

Other Options: For a hearty protein option Try Beyond Beef Crumbles®, or if you're a vegetarian like me, try diced browned Applegate® chicken apple sausage.

Egg Cups with Hot Smoked Salmon and Avocado-Chive Relish

You'll make 12 muffins

These egg cups are a fantastic portable breakfast that is light and easy to prepare. It also makes a good snack following an hour-long workout. This nutritious meal can be made with any kind of hot smoked salmon you might find on the grocery store shelves.

You can, for example, add sautéed mushrooms, sweet peppers, or diced kale.

12 eggs

¼ cup diced fresh basil

¼ cup crumbled goat cheese

1–2 cups fresh spinach or baby kale, diced

A dash of garlic powder

Some

¼ tsp

Pink salt or sea salt

8–10 gluten-free wraps made with rice or soy flour (I used Rudis tortillas)

About Salmon

Mix the basil, goat cheese, diced kale, and spices in a bowl.

Two muffin tins are sprayed with cooking spray. Tortilla wraps are ripped into thirds. The bottom of each muffin tin is covered with tortilla wraps. Each cup is nearly filled with salmon and, once filled, topped with some salmon. The tortilla wraps can extend past the height of each muffin hole. After filling each cup, a few pieces of salmon are added. Next, the cups are placed in the oven to bake for about 15 to 20 minutes or until a knife or toothpick inserted near the center of the muffin comes out clean and dry.

Chapter Two

With the Grain

Curried Garbanzo Beans with Eggplant and Brown Basmati Rice

Make a seafood stew with edamame and mung bean fettuccine

Three Citrus salad with pistachios and lemon dressing

Spicy

This recipe is my best ever garlicky croutons with super simple fast salad

Black Bean and Quinoa Pasta with Fresh Grilled Tomato, Basil, and Pine Nuts

Forbidden and delicious

Moroccan

Sauteed

Roasted beet salad with cannellini beans, and pistachio

With the Forbidden Food diet, you don't have to worry.

Swiss Chard and Artichoke Salad with Cannellini Beans and Bhutan Red Rice

Fast and Healthy Chicken Soup with Quinoa, Brown Rice, and Mushrooms

Roasted carrots and parsnips with Za'atar and forbidden rice.

Zesty and delicious!

Southern-Style

Vietnamese food

Makes 4 servings

Preheat the oven to 450 degrees

1 cup brown basmati rice

2.5 cups water or vegetable broth

1–2 teaspoons

Put one teaspoon of cumin seeds in your food (para 1)

Two medium eggplants medium eggplants, cut into ½-inch cubes and skins on

1 cup (approx) of onions

14-ounce can of fire-roasted tomatoes

1 15-ounce can garbanzo beans

Garlic

1/2 inch grated ginger root

1 Tablespoon of medium curry powder

1 Jalapeño pepper, seeded and minced

Pink salt and pepper can help

Garnish your workout with fresh cilantro.

Fresh

For the Rice:

Prepare 1 cup of steamed brown rice, adding 1 tablespoon of olive oil or canola oil. Heat skillet on medium-high and add about 2 tablespoons of cumin seeds. Once they begin to splutter, remove from heat. Add to rice and blend in, about 1/2 teaspoon of cumin.

For the Eggplant:

Toss lightly in olive oil and bake for about 20 minutes in a preheated oven. Once done, remove and set aside.

For the Curry:

“Heat” olive oil or butter in the skillet and sauté the onions.

Add in green bell peppers, tomatoes, garbanzo beans, garlic, ginger, and curry. Cook for about 2–3 minutes.

Add roasted eggplant and jalapeño pepper and continue cooking for about 10–15 minutes.

Serve family style, on a platter with the rice, with chopped fresh cilantro and lemon wedges.

Seafood Stew with Edamame and Mung Bean Fettuccine

Makes 6 servings

¼ cup extra virgin olive oil

2 medium onions, thinly sliced

2 tablespoons dried Greek oregano

1/2 teaspoon black pepper

⅛ teaspoon cayenne

4 teaspoons of red wine vinegar

½ cup white wine (optional)

Three cups vegetable stock or fish stock

Generous

3 cloves of garlic, smashed and minced

2 cans of tomatoes with garlic and basil (or plain)

In the summer of 2000, they ordered 2 pounds of fish fillets: orange roughy, mahi-mahi, black cod, scallops, and shrimp.

1 cup of torn curly kale (dinosaur kale), chopped into bite-sized pieces.

The Explore Asian® product comes with ½ package of edamame and mung bean fettuccine pasta.

The main ingredients for this dish include onions, olive oil, oregano, and cayenne pepper. Stirring them together in a large pot will produce a desired result.

After it has been reduced in volume and allowed to simmer for a while, add the stock, saffron, and garlic, and add the tomatoes. Bring to a boil.

Bring the liquid in the pot to a full boil; add the fish and kale to it. Reduce to low.

While that takes a while, cook pasta according to package instructions and set it aside.

Stir thoroughly and serve over cooked pasta.

For Crostini:

Keep your oven at 350 °F.

Cut slices of your favorite gluten-free multigrain bread into long strips. Then drizzle or brush with extra virgin olive oil. Add a pinch of sea salt or pink salt. Place the bread on a baking sheet and bake for about 15 to 20 minutes until crisp.

Three Leaf Salad with Pistachios and Lemon Dressing

Make it 2 servings

20–30 red seedless grapes

One

¾ (Cup) brown rice (or about 1½ cup cooked brown rice)

½ cup raw or roasted pistachios, chopped

About four tablespoons of chia seeds or flax seeds, or use hemp seeds.

A handful of each of these greens—or enough to make 2 salads:

Fresh baby spinach

Fresh basil leaves

How to make Fresh

Shallot vinaigrette

4 tablespoons

About shallots

1½ teaspoons honey

½ a teaspoon non-grainy honey mustard

3 tablespoons apple cider vinegar

2 tablespoons apple cider vinegar

2 large cloves of garlic minced

½ teaspoon onion granules

Grapes and Tomatoes:

In a large bowl, combine grapes and tomatoes with a a little olive oil. Serve in a small dish. Place the dish near a stove burner and watch them as they roast. Once done, remove and allow to cool.

A lot of foodies have a lot to say about how best to create a restaurant's original dish.

Black bean noodles with cabbage and a spicy peanut sauce

Makes 6 servings

Serve chilled

1

1 head cabbage, shredded 2 cabbage slaw mix

2 cups fresh sugar snap peas, or snow peas, sliced into half

½ cup shredded purple cabbage (about 1/2 head small cabbage)

One carrot package shredded carrots

Small cans Mandarin oranges and drained

1 ¼ to 1½ cups peanut sauce

4 teaspoons raw, unsalted sesame seed oil

Optional: Add ½ cup seasoned rice vinegar for extra tang

bunch cilantro, diced, including stems

1/2 cup

The pasta needed to be made using the package instructions, so it had to be cooled after boiling.

When making soup, boil the broccoli, carrots, and water. When the vegetables are cooled, shred the cabbage, and chop the carrots. Add the vegetable mixture to a large bowl and whisk in a peanut sauce, toasted sesame seed oil, and rice vinegar. Add noodles, and mix gently. Garnish

Serve it room temperature or chilled.

Garlic, Garlicky, best ever, garlicky croutons

For the Croutons:

Uses 2 cups of croutons

Preheat the oven to 350 degrees F.

¼ cup olive oil

3 to 4 good-sized cloves

4 to 5 slices of your favorite healthy bread, cut into one-inch cubes (not to exceed 1⅛ inches in diameter).

A, a few dashes of sea salt or pink salt

Optional: Add a teaspoon of dried Italian seasoning or herbes de' Provence.

For A Super Simple Fast Salad

Fresh smashed garlic

Extra virgin olive oil or pumpkin seed oil—yum!

Fresh squeezed lemon

Mix either baby greens or baby romaine lettuce

Radishes, sliced

Raw sunflower seeds

Store-bought rotisserie chicken or Applegate Farms® all natural turkey or chicken lunch meat

Prior to cooking the croutons, add the garlic to olive oil and allow to sit covered at room temperature for at least an hour or more. This will allow the olive oil to infuse with the peppery garlic. Believe me, it's worth the wait if you can leave it for even three hours.

In a large bowl, toss together the bread, olive oil, and salt and stir it several times in a circular motion.

Once coated with oil, sauté over medium heat for 4 to 6 minutes or until lightly browned. Add a few dashes of salt and a few cranks of fresh pepper and stir to coat. Place them on a cookie sheet to cool and crisped up. After that, serve on your salad.

To make this dish: Preheat the oven to 375 degrees F. In a large skillet over medium heat, heat 3 tablespoons of oil and heat a large saucepan filled with boiling water.

For a salad that's not just for kids or for your next holiday party, just smash some garlic with olive oil and squeeze in some fresh lemon, and mix thoroughly. Use baby lettuces, arugula, the radishes, a little raw sunflower seeds, and some croutons—or any kind of protein left over from cooking. If you want to make it a complete meal, I would add some leftover cooked chicken or turkey. I really like Applegate Farms®. Their chicken slices are just turkey slices, water, and spices!

Salsa

Make 4 servings

The Ancient Harvest® Gluten-Free Brown Rice Noodles are made with brown rice flour, organic potato starch, and whole wheat flour. With only 3 grams of net carbs per serving, Ancient Harvest® gluten-free noodles are good for those with special dietary needs, making them an easy way to enjoy pasta, pasta sauce, salad and more.

2 cups of tomatoes.

Sesame oil

1 box of Ancient Harvest® Bean and Quinoa elbow pasta

3–4 cloves

Two teaspoons of butter or ghee.

A cup of pine nuts

2–3 tablespoons of good quality parmesan cheese

About ½ cup goat cheese

2 teaspoon basil leaves, loosely chopped

Some ground black pepper

A pinch or two of pink salt or sea salt

To make a tasty snack, pour some olive oil in a bowl. Coat the tomatoes with the olive oil. Place on the rim of the baking sheet and roast them in a 350 degree oven until slightly blistered, about 15–20 minutes. You can

Cook noodles as per the package instructions.

In a large skillet, heat a drizzle of olive oil over medium-high. Add in garlic and stir quickly so garlic gets golden but does not burn. Remove the skins of the tomatoes and add the tomatoes, including their skins, to a skillet. Cook for about 2-3 minutes. Add in 2 teaspoons butter or ghee. Then stir in the pine nuts, cheeses, and fresh basil. Sometime add in a teaspoon of brown sugar

Forbidden Rice Salad, Heirloom Carrots, Cauliflower

Serves 6.

Serve this warm

Two cups vegetable broth

1 cup black rice or mahogany rice

2 tablespoons butter

1½ cups of cauliflower

2 heirloom carrots, slices into thin coins

1 large leek, sliced white

About ¼ bulb fennel, some fennel tops are kept aside

Extra-virgin olive oil or walnut oil

To taste

2½ teaspoons sumac

1 clove of garlic, minced

1 cup canned chickpeas, rinsed and drained

Ingredients: 1 teaspoon of Bragg's Liquid Aminos® Add 1 teaspoon to vegetables before roasting.

In a pot, bring hot water to a boil. Add rice to the hot water and covered soup pot. Reduce, add 2 tablespoons butter, cover, and simmer for about 25 minutes or until the rice is tender.

1. To make an exciting dish, cook cauliflower, carrots, leek, and fennel in a bowl. 2. Add a few pinches of salt and pepper. 3. Add some sumac and the garlic and stir to coat

Place vegetables in a pan and bake in the oven: about 15–20 minutes.

Once the vegetables are cooked, mix them with the chickpeas. Drizzle more olive oil in it and the skillet, then add in another vegetable stock or water, and sumac. Remove from heat, add in cauliflower and serve with chopped fresh fennel tops that's a bit of fresh black pepper.

Moroccan Rice with Beef, Dried Fruits, and Nuts

Makes 4–6 servings Preheat oven to 375 degrees F.

A 2-pound bag of baked red yam or 1-pound bag of diced red yam

A little extra virgin olive oil

1.5 pounds of round cut

1½ teaspoons allspice

a third of a teaspoon of cinnamon.

¼ teaspoon of cardamom, ground

3 tablespoons

1½ cups beef broth or water

¼ cup buckwheat, cooked

Four to five

Every 4–5 days, you should eat a small handful of dates.

two to three strips of lemon peel or pickled lemon

Mix it up with some spices and salt and pepper

2–3 teaspoons honey

¼–½ cup of pistachios, pine nuts or slivered almonds

A fresh, chopped mint, if available (optional)

For Red Yam

Roast the red yam in a pan with some olive oil and place it on a parchment paper-lined cookie sheet. Put in foil and make sure the oven is as hot as you can get the oven. Bake it for 25 minutes at 300 degrees to 350 degrees. Once cooked, remove and set aside.

For Beef and rice

Prepare small beef pieces in a large iron skillet. Once the meat is browned on all sides, add in the spices, broth, and the rice. Once the rice is tender, add in apricots, dates, lemon peel, yam, and honey. Let cook for about 25 minutes. Garnish with roasted almonds, mint, and honey. Serve.

Serve immediately!

Grilled miso and orange Tuna kabobs with mahogany rice

Makes 2–3 servings

This recipe requires marinating for up to 4 hours for best flavor.

For the Tuna:

Mix 3 tablespoons miso paste (or miso paste)

2 teaspoons of toasted sesame seed oil

1 tablespoon

1 table spoon orange juice

1 1/2 tablespoons coconut sugar or raw sugar.

2 teaspoons of fresh grated ginger

One teaspoon of orange

¼ teaspoon

Garlic 1 teaspoon

2 ahi tuna steaks cut into cubes

For the Rice:

¼ cup mahogany rice, or black rice

1 cup vegetable broth or chicken broth

For the Veggies:

two tablespoons sesame seed oil

2 raw cloves of garlic, smashed

3–4 carrots, julienne cut.

1 cup sugar snap peas, whole

4–5 green onions, trimmed

Dash or two of cayenne pepper

Sesame seeds

Add about ½ cup broccoli crowns.

Marinating the Ahi:

In a small sauce pan, combine miso paste, sesame seed oil, lime juice, orange juice, coconut sugar, fresh ginger, orange zest, cayenne pepper, and garlic. Over medium heat, mix marinade so that the sugar has dissolved and add marinade to a bowl or a bag, in which tuna steaks are placed. You can mix the bag or

Grilling the Kabobs:

Place the tuna on the grill. Let it sit for 5–10 minutes or until cooked.

Set the grill to medium-high and the burner to low to medium.

Carefully coat the grill surface with cooking spray, spraying at an angle. Add the skewers directly over heat and cook for about 4 – 5 minutes on each side. If you want perfectly cooked ahi steaks, cook for about 4 - 5 minutes on each side, or until the internal temperature reaches 145 degrees F. Remove

For the Rice:

In a small saucepan, bring broth and rice to a boil. Add broth to the rice and cook for about 20–25 minutes or until tender. Set aside.

For the Veggies:

Sesame seed oil is a good choice for cooking a Chinese vegetable dish because of its high smoking point. The oil is heated at high temperatures and garlic and other spices are quickly added. This dish will cook for only about 10-15 seconds. The quick cooking

Throw the vegetables on rice and top it with chicken kabob.

A Beet Salad with Cannellini Beans, Pistachio, Sorghum, and Goat Cheese

Make 6 servings

It has great texture and a slightly nutty flavor. It is a great hearty grain and can be a nice addition to salads and soups. You can make a great hot cereal by omitting the milk. It has been a staple for people in Africa for thousands of years. It is also called Milo by some brands.

2–3 cups of fresh beets, scrubbed and diced (about 6–8 beets).

Add 2 tablespoons olive oil

1 cup of vegetable broth

¼ cup cooked

2 cups cooked/1 can of cannellini beans

2 spoons of apple cider vinegar

You can roast your nuts or seeds.

Salt and pepper to taste

What to do

1/4 cup of fresh basil leaves, chopped rough

For the Beets:

Clean the beets by scrubbing them thoroughly, removing the stems, leaves, and any roots. Use a peeler to remove the skin. Cut the beets into little pieces, place them in a bowl, and then drizzle a little olive oil on top. Bake them on the middle rack in the oven. For about 30 minutes or until tender, they must be

For the Sorghum:

In a large saucepan over low heat, combine 2 cups of vegetable broth or low-sodium vegetable broth with 1/2 cup of sorghum. Bring to a boil. Reduce the heat to low. Cover and simmer for about 40–50 minutes until sorghum is tender. Do not let the soup boil out of the pan as you continue to make the salad

Assembling salad:

Toss all the veggies and spices together, except for the cheese and basil. Blend gently, adding more cheese or vinegar if you'd like. Serve in a bowl.

1. Don't cook the rice. It will be mushy and not taste like real food. 2. You can use cooked brown rice or cooked brown jasmine rice. 3. Buy the already cooked beets for a fast party or other event.

Forbidden Rice® Ramen shrimp and miso soup

Makes 2 servings

There are only certain things that require one to "be in a hurry for a fast meal?" Try out Lotus Foods forbidden rice ramen miso soup. That's only 4 minutes to cook and you can add other ingredients to keep the recipe easy to make.

2 package Lotus Foods® Forbidden Rice® Ramen with Miso Soup

6–8 large raw shrimp

How to cook spinach

2 cups water

About ½ teaspoon sriracha sauce or red chili and garlic paste

This dish is best made with medium-coarse sea snails that have been steamed and cleaned but that have not yet been shell-on. Once you have boiled the sea snails for 5 or 6 minutes, drain them and serve them with a sauce with added garlic. This dish would be eaten with rice noodles and has garlic in it.

Swiss chard and artichoke salad with cannellini beans and Bhutan red rice.

Swiss chard and artichoke salad

2 cups cooked Bhutan red rice.

One cup can of cooked cannellini beans

½ red bell pepper, seeded and diced

Halve a cup of kalamata olives.

12–14

6-8 large leaves of Swiss or rainbow chard, chopped

They have 10 marinated artichokes.

Pink salt, and fresh cracked black pepper to taste

Basil Dressing:

A ⅛-cup serving will make about ⅛ cup of dressing. If you wish, you can double the amount of dressing to make ¼ cup. You can store leftover dressing in the fridge

½ cup extra virgin olive oil.

2/3 of a heaping teaspoon tahini

Salt

Dash of cayenne

Fresh black pepper

6 tablespoon of lemon juice

1 teaspoon lemon zest

garlic, minced

6–8 fresh large basil leaves, chopped

Mix everything in the food processor--garlic, lemon, peppercorn, thyme. Taste it as you go along.

Throw all the salad ingredients into a mixing bowl. Squeeze lemon juice over them and toss to coat. Serve with more lemon if desired.

For added crunch, sprinkle the seeds into the bowl.

Chicken Soup

Makes 4–5 servings

1 32oz. package Pacific Free-Range Organic Chicken Broth®

2 carrots, diced

2 cloves garlic, finely chopped

One teaspoon of fresh thyme

Half a teaspoon of fresh herbs

¼ teaspoon of chopped rosemary

1 handfull

1 package of dried dried porcini mushrooms (or rehydrated)

1 whole rotisserie chicken, store-bought, fully cooked

1 cup marsala wine

2 8.5-ounce packages Brown Rice, Quinoa, and Lentil Packages (fully cooked in the grocery aisle)

1 chopped onion

Pink salt

Add all the ingredients into a large pot and heat it over high heat. Cook on low heat for about 10 minutes. Add all ingredients into the pot, and reduce heat to low-medium. It'll take about 3-5 minutes to cook through.

Clean chicken. Remove bones and skin. Boil pieces in water for 10-20 minutes and then add marsala wine and cook chicken further for about 10-20 minutes on low heat. Add cooked rice.

If you want to make your soup thicker and thicker, remove some of the carrots and blend in a food processor with some of the broth and add back into your soup. Also add more salt and pepper to taste.

Serve immediately.

Braised Carrots and Parsnips with Za'atar and Forbidden Rice

Makes 2–3 servings

The recipe includes a gluten-free substitute for soy sauce, which is a common condiment. As you use it, you'll get creative and come up with new uses for it. I use it to enhance other flavors, such as grilled chicken or fish, or to make dipping sauces like teriyaki and wasabi.

1 cup of vegetable broth

½ cup rice, forbidden.

½ pound Parsnips, peeled and cut into 2-inch pieces

½ pound carrots, peeled and cut into about 2-inch pieces

2 tablespoons

½ cup frozen edamame

2 Tablespoons of Za'atar Seasoning

1-2 teaspoons Bragg's Liquid Aminos

Pink salt and pepper to taste

In a saucepan, place 2 cups vegetable broth and 4 cups water. Bring to a boil. Reduce heat to low. Simmer for about 20 minutes or until water has evaporated and broth is thickened.

Mix cabbage, apples, parsnips and carrots in a bowl and drizzle with a little olive oil and season with a bit of fresh salt and pepper. Roast until the vegetables are tender or a little golden, stirring around halfway through coding.

As the main course of this recipe, I recommend you cook edamame in a bowl with a few tablespoons of water. You might want to cover the edamame with a paper towel, and you'll have to microwave them for 3 to 4 minutes.

This is a perfect salad to enjoy when you're on a vegetarian diet.

Makes about three servings

If you have been gluten free for years, you have tried quinoa, even if you are not gluten free. Kañiwa is just a smaller cousin to quinoa. Kañiwa doesn't need to be prewashed and it can be stored in your fridge for several days and you can cook it ahead of time and have it whenever you want. The quinoa itself is small and can be used for breakfast, lunch, lunch, dinner, etc.

For the Salad:

A handful of carrots, chopped (I used heirloom red and yellow carrots)

One cup fresh green beans

2 cups of water or vegetable broth

1 cup of kañiwa grain

Around 8–12 green Castelvetrano olives

½ pint grape tomatoes

6 fresh mozzarella pearls, cut into small pieces. Try these

1 cup of arugula

Extra-virgin olive oil or cooking oil

For the Basil Vinaigrette:

Makes about 1/2 cup of dressing

½ cup plus 2 tablespoons extra virgin olive oil

1 cup white balsamic vinegar

5 large garlic cloves, minced

15–18 large basil leaves, roughly chopped

Fresh cracked pepper

Pink salt

The Vegetables:

In large bowl, toss carrots green beans and tomatoes into the oven. Baste vegetables in oil, and roast for about 10–15 minutes, or until desired tenderness. Toss vegetables in bowl and serve. I like them slightly crunchy for this recipe.

The Kañiwa:

Heat broth, add salt, reduce heat, and simmer until it's absorbed by the grains—about 15 more minutes, stirring occasionally. Corn is ready when the germ of the grain can be seen. It must be stirred occasionally so as not to burn the corn.

Mix cooled brown rice with kañiwa beans, green beans, carrots, and olives. Add cracked black pepper. Then stir in tomatoes. Serve it on top of fresh arugula sprinkled with the extra dressing.

As the salad gets put together, the recipe provides tips for making the dressing as smooth and creamy as possible.

Castelvetrano olives are the dark green, oblong, creamy, and buttery olive. They are not fermented like many other olives, and retain their dark green appearance. Castelvetrano olives are often found in salad bars where other Mediterranean foods are located, or in jars in the

Healthy Southwestern Vegetarian Vegan soup with Bean and Quinoa pasta

Serves 8

½ to 1 cup of black beans (or about 1½ cups when cooked) and 1 cup of quinoa are just enough to make a whole meal.

2 chicken breasts, skinless, boneless, cut into cubes

4 cups of chicken broth

½ cup store-bought medium-spiced salsa

1 tablespoon extra virgin olive oil

2 medium onions, chopped

½ jalapeño pepper (more or less according to your taste)

A 15-ounce can of fire-roasted tomatoes in green chilies.

1½ cups tomato juice

2 or 3 medium carrots

2 tablespoons of freshly squeezed lime

1 cup (or 1/2 cup) fire-roasted corn

Three teaspoons of ground cumin

1 teaspoon medium chili powder

1 teaspoon of ancho powder (if you don't have it, add jalapeño and seeded diced)

1 teaspoon oregano

4 garlic cloves, smashed and minced

½ teaspoon

1½ cups chopped cilantro

medium zucchini or pattypan squash, or yellow squash, cut into ½-inch chunks.

Options:

Additional fresh cilantro

Dollop of plain Greek yogurt (or Mexican Crema)

Cook pasta according to package instructions

Combine the ingredients in a large pot and cover them over medium heat for 15–20 minutes over medium heat, stirring a few times occasionally. Then add zucchini and continue cooking for 5–8 minutes. Serve over pasta in a bowl and top with extra cilantro. If you want, add a dollop of nonfat Greek yogurt on top.

Garden Vegetables with Grilled Shrimp and Purple Yam Rice
Vietnamese Salad with Grilled Shrimp and Purple Yam

Makes 4 servings

10-14 pounds raw shrimp, shelled

½ cup, a serving of purple yam vermicelli (about 8 ounces)

1 cup carrots and 1 cup julienne sliced

1 cups (15 oz) fresh basil (or Thai basil), chopped

Mint

1 to 2 cups chopped cilantro

Onion

2–3 thinly sliced red Fresno peppers

(use green or red jalapeños instead)

4 tablespoons coarsely chopped unsalted roasted peanuts

For the Dressing:

½ cup brown sugar

cup of rice vinegar.

2-3 Tablespoons of red chili garlic paste

1 tablespoon of fresh lime juice

Two tablespoons fish sauce

1 tablespoon of sesame oil per head

1/2 cup of light soy sauce, if you are using vegetarian soy sauce

For the Shrimp:

You may start cooking your food by first heating your cast iron skillet on a high heat. Then add some cooking spray, and place your shrimp on the heat, turning it once, or until it is cooked.

For the Noodles:

If you are cooking pasta, you need to prepare the pot of water. Boil water in large pot on high heat. After boiling, add the pasta. Stir to separate the noodles and leave the pasta to stand for a few minutes or until the noodles are tender yet not soggy. Drain the pasta. Place the pasta into a bowl.

For the Dressing:

Mix the sugar with the rice vinegar to create a thick, sweet, tangy dressing. Then add this to a large bowl with the other dressing ingredients and stir well. Taste test the dressing and decide how much heat you want. If you want more tangy taste, add 1–2 more tablespoons of fresh lime juice.

Final Step:

After adding the pasta to the sauce, toss everything together. Add the roasted peppers to the top of the dish.

Chop 1/3 cup of peanuts and add to the top of the bowl. Garnish with peanuts and serve immediately after blending.

*If you are unable to find yam vermicelli, you may use thin rice noodles, but they should be the same amount of noodles as the original recipe. Cook them the same way as the recipe is written.

Chapter Three

Wraps, flatbreads, and pizzas

Grilled With Fire-Roasted Pepper and Goat Cheese

Mexican Wrap with Chicken and Chipotle Hummus

Take this lunch break.

Purple

Tuna and Lemony Artichoke Pizza with capers and Manchego cheese

Curry Salad Grapes Walnuts

Fast

French flatbread pizza

Buffalo Chicken Flatbreads | Chick-Fil-A | Pizza

Salmon

Fast Mediterranean open-faced sandwich.

Grilled Panini with Fire-Roasted Pepper and Goat Cheese

Makes 1 sandwich

Sandwiches can be a blessing and a curse to people who wish to eat healthy, as most people don't know the quality of ingredients in the sandwich, and the quantity of butter they use to grill it.

Why not make them at home instead?

Here are 2 things to try if you're making a quick panini

2 slices of your favorite multigrain or seeded gluten-free bread

a few slices of frozen grilled zucchini and eggplant, thawed with some homemade salsa.

A slice or two of roasted red pepper.

About an ounce of goat cheese, or your favorite low-fat cheese

Cracked pepper and sea salt or pink salt to taste

Butter, ghee, or Earth Balance® vegan spreads

Choices are: For more protein, add some slices of good all natural chicken or turkey.

Turn the skillet on medium-high heat.

Put a small amount of butter over the pan, then assemble the sandwich, add all the ingredients except butter and heat the pan. Once the sandwich is properly heated, flip it and brown the other side.

Eat.

Mexican Wrap: Tortilla Wrap with chicken and chipotle hummus

Makes enough for 2.

About 1 cup of rotisserie chicken, diced

¼ cup Kraft Singles®

1 Chipotle is in adobo sauce, chopped in a can in the ethnic section of the grocery store.

1 cup shredded cabbage (or 2 cups from the salad bar) 2. Combine the above ingredients, adding more vegetables as you wish Original: 2 cups 3. Add vinegar, brown sugar, and

½ mango, diced

¼ cup cilantro

Lime wedges

About ½ cup store-bought red pepper hummus (or plain hummus)

The If you're looking for an article rewriter, then a free alternative is called My Article Rewriter. It's not the same functionality

Mix together Vegenaise, a little of the sauce from a can of chipotle in adobo, shredded cabbage, diced mango, cilantro, squirts of lime, and a dash of salt. Toss gently, but avoid over doing.

Add the other half of the chipotle and hummus to the small mixing bowl. Mix thoroughly.

Mix the avocado with the chicken and slaw mixture. Add toasted wrap. Add slices of cucumber, red onion, and a squeeze of lime. Enjoy.

It's an easy and tasty dish that's delicious.

Serve this to everyone

About

two to teaspoons

¼ cup cilantro

About 4 teaspoons purple onion, minced

1 small ataulfo mango diced

2 gluten-free tortillas

2–4 butter lettuce leaves or romaine lettuce

2 to 3 teaspoons Hot Curry Paste

Not optional: ½ red bell pepper, diced

If you have any leftover yams or sweet potatoes, you can toss those in with the chicken.

Cook up some store-bought rotisserie chicken and add Vegenaise® to the mix

In a medium bowl combine the eggplant relish with Vegenaise®. Add cilantro, purple onion and chicken and stir well but do not break up the chicken. Add mango and add a dash of salt if desired.

Place the tortilla wrap in a skillet, and add a little cooking spray; ghee, or oil to the pan.

Remove the rolls individually, placed them on plates.

Add 2-3 lettuce leaves onto the tortilla wrap.

Divide the chicken curry into two equal portions and place them on top of the lettuce.

Serve open or rolled

Add some of the vegenaise to the tortilla before you add some of the lettuce and chicken.

If you can't find a ripe mango, then just pass on it. Frozen mangoes are devoid of all flavor. * A: The idea is to paraph

** The best eggplant relish I can find is Patak Binjal Eggplant Relish®, which is widely available in many grocery stores. I use it to substitute for mild curry paste.

Purple Cauliflower Pizza with Sundried Tomatoes and Cilantro Pesto

Makes 2 9-inch pizza crusts

Cauliflower can be found in red, yellow, green, and purple. Most people find them to taste about the same, but it's fun to have different food colors in your cooking.

For the Crust:

4 cups cauliflower, grated or chopped fine

Two

1 ¼ cups shredded part-skim mozzarella cheese

cup parmesan cheese (or pecorino romano)

A half-teaspoon of dried oregano

Cook 1 tablespoon chickpea flour

½ teaspoon garlic powder

A few pinches of pink salt and pepper, now that's tasty

For the Toppings:

3–4 medallions of goat cheese.

1 cup sun-dried tomatoes (packed in olive oil)

½ cup Kalamata olives

In ¼ teaspoon, crushed red pepper flakes

For the Cilantro Pesto

You can make about 1 cup

1 bunch of cilantro

½ cup of olive oil.

half a cup of pine nuts or walnuts, roughly chopped

2 large cloves of garlic

Use one lemon

Salt and pepper to taste

Add a bit of cayenne

Place parchment paper on a rimmed baking sheet or on a cookie sheet.

Grate the florets and cut into small pieces. Place a large bowl with the grated cauliflower, and cover with a paper towel. Microwave on high power for about three minutes, or until the cauliflower steams. Stir and cook for a few minutes or until soft. Remove and allow to cool

In a bowl, combine the egg, mozzarella, and Parmesan cheese. Then mix in the cauliflower, oregano, chickpea flour, and garlic powder until the ingredients are well distributed. After mixing, have half of the egg and cheese mixture ready for baking, while the other half can be refridgerated for later. In one layer on a baking sheet, flatten the

Top pizza with the goat cheese, Kalmaata olives, and sun-dried tomatoes. Cook for about 10–12 minutes or until the edges of the crust begin to brown, then add the cilantro pesto.

For the Pesto:

In a food processor, combine all ingredients into a smooth, paste-like consistency. To create the right consistency for a drizzle, use a plastic squeeze bottle.

Tuna with Lemony Artichoke Pizza and Capers and Manchego cheese

Makes 2 flatbread pizzas

Marinated artichokes, drained and sliced in half

About 4–6 teaspoons manchego cheese, grated, or Parmesan Cheese

A dash of red chili flakes would be perfect.

2 teaspoons minced garlic

Have a drink of water with lemon wedges

1 spoon of extra virgin olive oil

2 gluten-free tortilla wraps

Tongol Tuna can be packed in either water or oil, drained or Tonnino.

2–3 teaspoons capers

6–7 Pitted olives, chopped, look for them on the salad bars. They are bright greenish blue.

Dash of red pepper

Fresh cracked pepper

Microgreens

Optional: finely sliced purple onion

Garlic, basil, or a combination of both to garnish

The artichokes are taken out of the refrigerator and placed on a cutting board. A food processor is then used to add lemon juice, red chili flakes, garlic, a nice pinch or two of pink salt, and black pepper; the mixture is pulsed at least 2 or 3 times, until only just blended, then olive oil is added and the mixture is pulsed for a few

Chop onion and place in a bowl. Add in lemon, if using. Season with lemon, salt, and pepper.

Place 2 tortilla wraps on a baking tray with the inside of the tortillas coated with cooking spray. Cover the tortilla with the artichoke mixture, then sprinkle tuna, capers, and olives on top. Add any remaining artichokes on top.

Bake in the oven for about 20–25 minutes and top with microgreens or other small chopped greens.

Serve warm.

Curried Goat Cheese and Green Apple Salad with Grapes and Walnuts

Makes enough for 2–3 wraps. Preheat oven to 350 degrees F.

1 small to medium sweet green potato

2 large sweet green potato

2 sweet potato 3

small to medium potato

2 teaspoons extra virgin olive oil

Add some salt to taste

6 teaspoons mild curry powder (or use Patak's® mild curry paste)

3-4 teaspoons of mayonnaise

2-4 tablespoons yogurt.

½ diced granny apples (skins can stay on if desired)

About ½ cup slivered almonds or walnuts, chopped

Get your grape intake for the day

2–3 gluten-free tortilla wraps

Optional: Fresh cilantro or frozen, thawed peas added in

Boil a couple of potatoes in a pot of water. Drain, place them in a bowl, cover with olive oil, a pinch of salt, and stir. Make sure the potatoes are coated in oil. Put a sheet of aluminum foil over the pot and bake for 15–20 minutes (without a cover) or until they are just tender because they shouldn't be mushy.

While the yam is cooking, combine the precooked quinoa and brown rice mixture with the sauce and mix thoroughly.

Add a few drops of vegetable oil. Add Greek yogurt, apples, almonds, and grapes together and stir gently.

Once the Yams are done, they should be removed from the oven and allowed to cool.

Make a mixture of ingredients by mixing the spices, oil, and salt in a bowl. If desired, add cilantro and/or peas.

Place tortillas on a plate and roll them up.

You can also make extra-sauce by mixing yogurt, curry paste, and Vegenaise® and serve a dollop on the side with each wrap.

Chicken wrap Red Pepper Hummus

Serve your meal cold

2 gluten-free tortilla wraps

¼ cup of store-bought hummus

Eat carrots and get shredded carrots from the salad bar.

About this recipe.

One or two tablespoons banana peppers

A 5-8 slice of all natural chicken lunch meat from an organic source.

Peas, broccoli, or any kind of your choice

3–4 Tablespoons mayonnaise or vegenaise

Lettuce or other salad leaves of choice

To add spice, combine some Harissa with the red pepper hummus.

Place a tortilla, spread on with a red pepper hummus.

To make a chicken salad wrap, add shredded carrots, purple onion and banana peppers. Add slices of chicken and drizzle some mayonnaise (or your preferred condiment) on top. Add a little bit of salt and pepper. Add some fresh sprouts on

Thai flatbread pizza with shrimp and peanut sauce

Make 2 flattedbread pizzas

Start your meal with cabbage coleslaw

1 teaspoon olive oil.

About the ingredients in this recipe

A few slivers of purple onion

8 medium shrimp

One to two teaspoons soy sauce

2 tortilla wraps

About

1–2 tablespoons of almonds, cashews or peanuts, chopped

1–3 tablespoons fresh cilantro, chopped

2–3 tsp of sesame seeds

For the Slaw:

3 cups shredded red and white cabbage

About 3 tablespoons Vegenaise® or mayonnaise or mayonnaise

Dash of cayenne pepper

Dash or two of pink salt

1 tablespoon

Three to four tablespoons of cilantro, roughly chopped

For the flat bread pizzas:

In a small skillet, heat sesame seed oil until it is very hot. Add in peppers and onions which then are cooked for about three minutes and are stirred often. Add in cooked (but raw) shrimp and cook for a minute.

Use a cookie sheet to cook your Mexican shrimp tacos.

Put the pot with the chicken, onion, and ginger into the oven. Allow it to cook for 20-25 minutes. Then top with sesame seeds, cilantro, and peanuts.

Include Asian slaw on your plate.

For the Slaw:

Combine the ingredients together and serve.

Makes about 2 cups of slaw (enough for 2 servings).

Buffalo Chicken - Flatbread Pizza

Make two personal-sized pizzas

This recipe can be tailored to fit with whatever is available at your local supermarket, but no matter what, it's a great, quick meal for lunch or dinner. The kids will love it!

4 chicken breasts, fully cooked

2 flatbreads are the bread of choice when making a PB&J.

The key to a well-designed program is the purple onion (4% carbohydrate).

About ½ cup crumbled blue cheese or goat cheese

Louisiana is often served at parties. However, it can also be enjoyed on its own.

Fresh cilantro, chopped

For the Chicken:

Make homemade chicken nuggets by cutting up your favorite grilled chicken breast. Mix extra virgin olive oil and seasoning together. Spray a baking sheet with cooking spray, pile the chicken seasoned, then coat it with cooking spray. Be careful not to overcook them; when they go from golden brown to blackened.

Cook it

For the Pizza:

Place your flatbread or tortilla on a greased baking sheet.

Prepare pasta by mixing egg, flour, salt, and cheese. Cook for about 12 minutes or until the onions begin to brown and the cheese starts to melt. Add the sauce and serve.

Top a salad with a combination of avocado, lime zest or lemon juice and serve immediately.

Chicken Salad Wrap with Honey Mustard Slaw and Black Risotto

Makes 2 servings and is great served cold or at room temperature

½ cup black rice or mahogany rice blend (look for Lundberg japonica)

1 cup of water or vegetable broth

It can be anything cooked -- chicken, turkey, fish, pork, etc. It can be completely prepared and ready to eat or it can be just raw. For example, you can have

2 teaspoons lemon juice

1 tablespoon extra virgin olive oil

Add salt and pepper to taste

¾ teaspoon sumac

1 minced garlic clove

½ cup thinly sliced green onion

About

Add two tablespoons of cilantro, chopped.

1 teaspoon fresh mint, chopped

½⁄1 teaspoon lemon or lime zest

3 tablespoons slivered almonds or pistachio

You can also add your favorite store-bought hummus to the tortilla. It will help to make the salad taste even better.

In a small saucepan, combine the ingredients over high heat. Bring to a boil, then reduce heat and simmer about 30–45 minutes or until tender.

Drain excess water if needed. Allow to cool uncovered.

Cook the chicken in a large bowl with lemon, olive oil, salt, pepper, mustard, garlic and sumac. Let stand about 5 minutes.

After the rice has been stirred in along with the remaining ingredients, gently stir.

To this day, the taco is thought of as a Mexican dish, despite the fact that it evolved in the United States. Now, you can enjoy tacos as you wish: with or

Fast Open-Faced Mediterranean Wrap

Makes 4 servings

The dish is a delicious pasta wrap with pesto, feta, lemon, green or black olives, pine nuts, cherry tomatoes, green or black arugula, shredded baby spinach and shredded rotisserie chicken.

2 teaspoons extra-virgin olive oil

½ cup

About lemons

1 teaspoon lemon zest

One tablespoon of red wine vinegar.

1 teaspoon extra virgin olive oil

2 cloves garlic

½ teaspoon dry oregano (or half teaspoon if it's fresh)

Three to four handfuls flat-leaf parsley, minced

5 cups fully cooked grains, cooked in water or broth, cooled

What it includes:

About 2 cups skinless boneless diced chicken

½ cucumber, diced

A ½ cup of Kalamata olives, pitted, diced

About 2–4 cups of chopped rainbow chard or kale

quarter cup peppers

1/4 cup crumbled feta cheese

Make your dressing salty and spicy

2 tortilla wraps

Add about a teaspoon of sesame oil. Stir the sesame oil and salt into the pine nuts, and cook until golden brown, about 7-10 minutes. If skillet is getting too hot, rotate skillet while working on it. Note : Do not use salted or smoked pine nuts.

To make the dressing: In a large bowl, mix together the lemon juice, lemon zest, red wine vinegar, olive oil, garlic, oregano, green onions, parsley, pink salt, and black pepper. Add diced chicken and allow it to marinate for several minutes

Put all the ingredients, except for tortilla wraps, in a bowl and mix together gently.

Modify to taste.

Create easy dinner options, like taco or burrito wraps, or simply get a snack on its own, without the wrap.

Fast and Easy: Sea-Er-A Tuna with Edamame and Mung Bean Fettucine with Peanut Sauce and Sugar Snap Peas

Kabocha Squash, Gnocchi, and Sage

Zucchini

Pasta

Edamame

Mushroom Soup with carrots and bhutan red rice

Mexican Chicken with Penne and Peppers

Easy Paella

Mexican Black Bean Stack with Vegetables, Red Quinoa, and Brown Rice

Chicken and Asparagus served with sun-dried tomatoes and mushrooms

"Fast and easy": seared tuna, edamame and mung bean fettuccine.

Make enough for 2 people.

One or two tuna steaks

A little bit of sesame seed oil

1½ cups

1 cup snowpeas

¼ cup

Halve red bell pepper

3 spring onions, chopped

About ½ cup (or more) of this Thai Peanut Sauce and your goals!

Optional: chop and sprinkle with cilantro or peanuts.

Prior to cooking tuna, allow for about 10 minutes at room temperature.

Drizzle sesame oil on the top of tuna before grilling to prevent it from burning. You can do this directly on the grill.

Grilling or frying a tuna steak requires heat, which in turn, requires an element. The temperature of the element determines how well the tuna gets cooked.

Once you've finished, allow to rest

In a medium pot, bring about 3 cups of water to a boil. Add 3 cups of fettuccine. Reduce heat and simmer gently for about 7–8 minutes or until the pasta is cooked through.

Once rinsed, drain and wash with cold water.

Mix the tuna with 1-tablespoon toasted sesame oil and use to cook with a few vegetables until the vegetables start getting tender. Then add in the noodles and the Thai Peanut Sauce and stir to coat. Divide to two plates and serve.

Break the tuna steaks into pieces and spread them out on top of the noodles, vegetables, and other toppings. Top with cilantro, sesame seeds, or chopped peanuts.

CPSIA information can be obtained
at www.ICGtesting.com
Printed in the USA
LVHW060216160722
723616LV00015B/806

9 781804 768624